MELANOMA CANCER DIET COOKBOOK

A DIETARY GUIDE FOR WELLNESS AND RESTORATION

BY

Angel B. Maurice

Table of Contents

Introduction

Our resilience and fortitude are often tested and refined in times of difficulty. When people are given the news that they have melanoma, they begin a journey that will test not only their physical strength, but also their willingness to take on the difficulties of life head-on. As the worst form of skin cancer, melanoma necessitates bravery, resiliency, and a comprehensive strategy for treatment. Nutrition, the foundation of health, is an integral part of this comprehensive approach.

Hello, and thank you for taking the time to learn more about "Nutrition Strategies for Melanoma Warriors: A Cookbook for Health and Healing." More than just a compilation of recipes, this cookbook is a moving testament to the role that food can play in the battle against melanoma. Here, we'll discuss how the foods we eat can help or hurt our efforts to maintain a healthy lifestyle.

Without prompt diagnosis and treatment, melanomas are a dangerous foe that can quickly spread. Its journey often includes operations, chemotherapy, immunotherapy, and radiation, and it affects countless people and their families. Nutritional support for melanoma patients is crucial and should not be overlooked in place of medical treatment.

The road to recovery from melanoma can be tough, with physical and mental health being tested by treatment side effects. Many difficulties can arise for patients, including a lack of appetite, weariness, nausea, and altered taste perception. The foods in this cookbook are meant to nourish, comfort, and maintain you through these trying times.

The Meaning of Melanoma

It's important to know who we're up against before we start cooking. Melanin is the pigment that gives our skin, hair, and eyes their color, and melanoma develops in the cells that make it. While the skin is the most common site of onset, the eyes and mucous membranes are not immune.

Melanoma is particularly dangerous because it can metastasize to other organs, including the lymph nodes, lungs, liver, and brain. Regular skin examinations and consultations with a dermatologist are necessary for people at risk because early detection and fast treatment are vital in slowing its spread.

Many factors, including genetics, UV exposure, and immune system performance, contribute to the development of melanoma. We may not be able to change our genetic make-up, but we can take preventative measures like using sunscreen and eating well to reduce the risk of skin cancer.

Nutrition as a Therapeutic Strategy for Melanoma

This cookbook is meant to be a supportive resource for people coping with melanoma; it is not intended to replace professional medical care. Our immunological response, inflammatory levels, and vitality are all affected by the foods we eat on a molecular level. Consequently, melanoma sufferers can benefit greatly from utilizing the power of nutrition to aid with their treatment and recovery.

In the following chapters, you'll find an abundance of recipes, meal plans, and nutritional insights developed specifically for melanoma patients and their needs. We'll talk about the anti-inflammatory advantages of certain foods, the restorative effects of antioxidant-rich fare, and how to put together well-rounded, healthy meals. This cookbook includes a wide variety of recipes for breakfast, lunch, dinner, and even dessert that are all healthy and delicious.

Although battling melanoma is difficult, it can be a catalyst for personal development and positive change. Keep in mind that nutrition is a potent ally as you move forward on your journey. We're going to go on a foodie excursion together that will do more than just satisfy your stomach. You have entered a realm where tasty remedies abound.

Chapter 1

We Lay the Groundwork

Knowledge is your first and most powerful weapon in the fight for health and wellness. Building a solid nutritional foundation is essential before beginning a journey toward healing when fighting melanoma. This section will act as a roadmap, arming you with the information you need to make nutritional decisions that will benefit your health as you fight melanoma.

Guidelines for Melanoma Patients' Dietary Maintenance

It is important to grasp the fundamentals of nutrition before delving into the specifics of a melanoma-friendly diet. You don't have to be a melanoma sufferer to benefit from these guidelines for eating well.

Nutritional Balance: A healthy diet contains all the essential nutrients for optimal bodily function. It's important to get enough of everything, from carbs and proteins to fats and minerals. All of these factors contribute to your health in their own way.

While the quality of your food is essential, the quantity you eat is also important. As some melanoma therapies might cause weight changes, gaining weight due to overeating may not be desirable. Controlling your portions is an effective strategy for managing your weight and stamina.

Adequate hydration is essential for good health but is frequently disregarded. Hydration aids in the evacuation of toxins, aids digestion, and keeps the body's fluid levels stable.

If your immune system is weak from treatment, it is extremely important to follow good food safety procedures. Fruits and vegetables should be washed thoroughly, raw meats should be avoided, and unpasteurized dairy products should be treated with caution.

Foods high in dietary fiber, like whole grains, fruits, and vegetables, are important for digestive health. They are useful for avoiding the side effects of constipation that some drugs can cause.

Restrict your intake of sugary and highly processed foods as much as possible. These can cause energy highs and lows and are linked to a possible worsening of inflammation.

Treat yourself occasionally, but don't make it a habit. While it's important to pay attention to what your body needs, it's also nice to treat yourself every once in a while.

Essential Healing Nutrients

Now that we've established that proper nutrition is essential for people with melanoma, let's look more closely at which nutrients are most crucial.

Protein: Protein is essential for immune system health and tissue repair. Include lean protein sources in your diet such as poultry, fish, beans, and tofu. Small, protein-rich meals and snacks might help you keep your muscle mass even if you lose your appetite while undergoing treatments.

Fatty fish like salmon and flaxseeds are good sources of omega-3 fatty acids, which have anti-inflammatory effects. During therapy for melanoma, they may help lessen inflammation.

Antioxidants are chemicals in fruits and vegetables that stave off cell damage from free radicals. Antioxidants include vitamins C and E, as well as selenium and beta-carotene. Some of the best food sources are berries, citrus fruits, nuts, and seeds.

The vitamin D in milk helps maintain healthy bones and immune systems. Vitamin D can be synthesized through exposure to sunlight, but if you're worried about getting too much sun, your doctor may recommend taking a supplement instead.

Strong bones and teeth can only be maintained with a diet rich in calcium. Calcium can be found in dairy, leafy greens, and soy or almond milk that has been fortified.

Folate is a type of vitamin B that helps with DNA replication and damaged cells can be repaired.

Iron: Iron is necessary for carrying oxygen throughout the body. Iron levels can be kept stable by eating foods like lean meats, legumes, and iron-fortified cereals.

Zinc: Helps with immunity and mending wounds. Zinc can be found in foods including almonds, dairy, and lean meats.

Foods high in dietary fiber promote digestion and may alleviate the common side effects of treatment-related constipation. You can obtain a lot of fiber from eating whole grains, fruits, vegetables, and beans.

Keep in mind that your specific dietary requirements may change as you progress through your melanoma treatment. It is crucial to coordinate your nutrition plan with your healthcare providers and a trained dietitian so that it complements your condition and treatment. To make sure you're getting the vitamins and minerals you need for recovery and vitality, they can provide you with individualized advice and track your progress.

In the next chapters, we'll go deeper into how these dietary guidelines can be used to whip up healing meals that taste great. We'll give you a wide variety of dishes that are tailored to your preferences and diet, from stimulating breakfasts to hearty dinners and even delicious desserts. With our combined efforts, we can turn food into a potent weapon in your fight against melanoma.

Chapter 2

Melanoma Survivors' Meal Planning

Knowing what to eat while undergoing melanoma treatment is only half the battle;

careful meal preparation is also essential. A well-planned diet can be a potent weapon in the fight against melanoma by supplying your body with the nutrition it needs to recover and thrive. Here, we'll delve into the science and practice of planning and preparing nutritious meals that will give you the energy and stamina to take on each day.

Making Well-Rounded, Nutritious Dishes

Your quest for optimal health begins and ends with a focus on nutritional balance. Maintaining your health and providing your body with the fuel it needs during treatment depends on the nutrients you get from the food you eat. The fundamentals of healthy eating are broken down here:

Consume a rainbow's worth of colors by incorporating a wide range of fruits and vegetables into your daily diet. Antioxidants and nutrients are commonly represented by their respective colors. Beta-carotene is abundant in orange and yellow fruits and vegetables, whereas vitamin and mineral content is high in greens.

Power up with protein at every meal by eating lean protein. Protein is crucial for immune system health and the repair of damaged tissues. You can't go wrong with options like skinless chicken, fish, tofu, beans, and lentils.

Avocados, almonds, seeds, and olive oil are all examples of healthy fats that you should incorporate into your diet. These fats aid in nutrition absorption and are beneficial to general health.

Choose whole grains over refined ones whenever you can. Brown rice, quinoa, and whole wheat pasta are examples of whole grains that are higher in fiber and minerals.

If you eat dairy products or substitutes, go for the low- or no-fat varieties. Choose almond or soy milk that has been fortified if you prefer a dairy-free diet.

Avoid overeating by keeping track of how much food you put on your plate. If your treatment is causing you to lose your appetite, try eating more frequently and in smaller portions.

Smart snacking means always having something healthy on hand, like a handful of nuts, some yogurt, or a piece of fruit. These are an easy method to keep your energy up all day long.

Timing Meals and Portion Control

Meal planning, and specifically portion control, is crucial when undergoing treatment for melanoma. Due to treatment-related appetite loss, it may be difficult to consume normally-sized meals. To help you control your portion sizes, here are some suggestions:

Try eating more frequently and in smaller portions throughout the day instead of three large meals. Even if your appetite is low, this can help you acquire the nutrients your body needs.

Focus on how your body tells you when it's hungry or full. If you're not hungry, there's no need to eat everything on your plate.

Eat off of smaller dishes and bowls to save waste. This trick can make your dish look more substantial, which can aid in portion management.

When you eat mindfully, you focus on the present moment and really take in the tastes and sensations of your food. This can help you feel full after eating less.

When it comes to meal preparation, time is just as important as the meals themselves. The timing and frequency of your meals have an effect on your vitality, digestion, and health as a whole.

1.Consistent Meal Times: Try to create regular meal times to assist in regulating your body's internal clock. Consistency can also make it easier to manage medications and treatment schedules.

2.Preparation Is Key: Plan your meals and snacks ahead of time. This can prevent the stress of having to figure out what to eat when you're already hungry.

3.Post-Treatment Meals: If you're suffering side effects like nausea, prepare lighter meals for after your treatment sessions. Simple, readily digestible foods like rice, bread, or yogurt can be comforting.

4.Stay Hydrated: Include liquids like water, herbal teas, or hydrating smoothies throughout the day to maintain optimum hydration levels.

Remember that meal planning is a flexible process that may be tailored to your specific needs and interests. It's vital to work with your healthcare team and a certified dietitian to personalize your meal plan to your unique treatment regimen and any dietary limitations you may have.

In the future chapters, we'll delve into the intricacies of melanoma-fighting nutrients and give you with a broad selection of recipes tailored to your nutritional needs. Together, we'll construct meals that fuel your body, support your healing journey, and offer warmth and happiness to your table.

Chapter 3

Melanoma-Fighting Ingredients

In our endeavor to harness the power of nutrition in the battle against melanoma, understanding the specific components that can promote your body's resistance is of critical importance. Foods high in antioxidants, anti-inflammatory substances, and immune-boosting nutrients are discussed in this chapter as potential melanoma-fighting elements that can play an important part in your recovery.

Foods High in Antioxidants

Protecting cells from damage and inflammation caused by oxidative stress is the job of antioxidants, which the body produces naturally. Antioxidant-rich meals are highly beneficial for melanoma sufferers since they help fight free radicals and inflammation.

Antioxidants like anthocyanins and vitamin C abound in berries like blueberries, strawberries, raspberries, and blackberries. These chemicals have been shown to reduce oxidative stress on cells.

Vitamin C, a potent antioxidant that helps maintain a healthy immune system and beautiful skin, is abundant in citrus fruits like oranges, grapefruits, and lemons.

Greens like spinach, kale, and Swiss chard are rich in anti-inflammatory phytonutrients and the antioxidant vitamins A, C, and K.

Foods high in antioxidant vitamin E and healthful fats can be found in nuts and seeds such as almonds, walnuts, flaxseeds, and chia seeds.

Flavonoids, antioxidants found in dark chocolate with a high cocoa content, have been shown to benefit heart health and provide for a satisfyingly sweet treat without the need for refined sugars.

Green tea, as well as herbal teas like chamomile and peppermint, are great beverage options since they contain large amounts of antioxidants.

Foods That Reduce Inflammation

The harmful effects of melanoma might be compounded by the body's chronic inflammation. The use of anti-inflammatory foods can aid in the control of inflammation and the maintenance of general health.

Anti-inflammatory omega-3 fatty acids are abundant in fatty fish like salmon, mackerel, and sardines. These lipids have anti-inflammatory and heart-healthy properties.

Curcumin, turmeric's main ingredient, is a powerful anti-inflammatory. It can be used to impart a comforting, earthy taste to dishes like soups and stews by adding curry powder.

Similar to ginger, ginger is an anti-inflammatory spice. It's great for cooking and also makes a calming tea when steeped in hot water.

Olive oil is an excellent source of healthful fat, especially extra virgin olive oil, which includes chemicals that have anti-inflammatory benefits. It works wonderfully in salad dressings and sautés.

Lycopene, a type of carotenoid with anti-inflammatory properties, is abundant in tomatoes. The antioxidant lycopene in tomatoes can be made more readily available by cooking them.

Berries: Not only are they high in antioxidants, but they also have chemicals that can aid in reducing inflammation.

Ingredients That Boost Your Immunity

In the battle against melanoma, a robust immune system is essential. You can strengthen your body's defenses with the help of these immune-enhancing chemicals.

Allicin, a chemical found in garlic, has antibacterial and immune-boosting qualities. Spice up your savory foods with garlic and boost your immune system at the same time.

Yogurt and probiotics: a strong immune system is tied to a healthy digestive tract. Yogurt and other probiotic-rich foods like kefir can keep your gut microbiota in check.

Vitamin C, which has been shown to have beneficial effects on the immune system, is abundant in citrus fruits.

Mushrooms: Compounds found in mushrooms like shiitake and maitake have been shown to improve immunological response. You can use them to enhance the flavor of soups and stir-fries.

Foods high in lean protein, such as lean poultry, fish, and tofu, are good for the immune system because they contain important amino acids.

Vegetables with vibrant colors, such as bell peppers, carrots, and sweet potatoes, are packed with immune-supporting vitamins and minerals.

You don't have to give up taste or diversity to incorporate these melanoma-fighting substances into your diet. They add nutritional value and aesthetic appeal to your meals.

You'll find delicious new uses for these staples as you peruse the recipes in this booklet. You may help nourish your body and aid in your recovery by including foods like antioxidant-rich berries in your morning smoothie, aromatic turmeric-spiced dishes, and delightful meals with omega-3-rich salmon.

It's important to tailor your diet to your specific demands and treatment goals. Creating a personalized nutrition strategy that best supports your melanoma treatment and recovery is best done in collaboration with your healthcare team and a qualified dietitian. In the next chapters, we'll explore specific dishes that highlight the power of these melanoma-fighting foods, ensuring that your path to health is both delicious and rewarding.

Chapter4

Recipes for the Morning Meal

As the first meal of the day, breakfast is a great chance to fuel up for the day ahead. These dishes are meant to be both satisfying and energizing, providing a solid foundation for the day ahead. We have something tasty for everyone, whether they want something fast and simple or a leisurely weekend brunch.

Recipe for a Refreshing Morning Smoothie

Ingredients:

One cup of berries (such as blueberries, strawberries, or raspberries) either fresh or frozen One ripe banana half a cup of Greek yogurt (or a dairy-free substitute) a tablespoon of chia seeds a cup of unsweetened almond milk (or any milk of your choice)Sweeten to taste with honey or maple syrup (optional); serve over ice (also optional).

Instructions:

Put everything in a blender and blend until smooth.

2. Add ice cubes if you want a colder consistency, and blend until smooth and creamy.

3. If you want it sweeter, taste it and add honey or maple syrup.

4. Pour into a glass, and savor your wholesome morning smoothie.

Bowl of Quinoa for Breakfast

Ingredients:Ingredients: 1/2 cup quinoa; 1 cup water; 1/2 cup sliced strawberries; 1/4 cup blueberries; 1/4 cup chopped nuts (such as almonds, walnuts, or pecans); 1 tablespoon honey or maple syrup; 1/2 teaspoon cinnamon; pinch salt

Instructions:

First, you should give the quinoa a good cold water rinse. Second, start boiling some water in a pot. Put in a pinch of salt and the quinoa you just rinsed. To cook the quinoa, cover the pot, lower the heat to low, and let it simmer for 15 to 20 minutes.

4. Use a fork to fluff the quinoa and place it in a bowl.

5Add sliced strawberries, blueberries, and chopped almonds to the cooked quinoa.

Six, finish it off with some honey, maple syrup, and cinnamon.

Seventh, stir everything together and eat your healthy quinoa breakfast dish.

Poached egg on avocado toast (3)

Ingredients:

2 slices of gluten-free bread or whole-grain bread• 1 avocado, ripe

ingredients:

2 large eggs, salt, and pepper to taste, red pepper flakes (optional)• Chopped fresh herbs (such as cilantro, parsley, or chives)

Instructions:

1. Toasted the bread until it was the crispness you liked. Cut the ripe avocado in halves, remove the pit, and scoop the flesh into a bowl as the bread toasts.

With a fork, mash the avocado and season it with salt and pepper to taste.

Third, poach the eggs by bringing water to a simmer in a saucepan. Separate the eggs into individual bowls after cracking. Make a small whirlpool in the water by stirring it with a spoon while it's cooking. Gently place one egg into the vortex's core. If you like a runnier yolk, poach for 3–4 minutes; if you prefer a firmer yolk, poach for longer. Replace the second egg and carry on.

4. Smear the mashed avocado on the toasted bread slices in an equal layer.

5. Top each piece of avocado toast with a poached egg. Add more salt, pepper, and crushed red pepper if you want it spicy.

7. Top with a few sprigs of fresh herb. Immediately after cooking the egg, top the avocado toast with the egg and serve.

Chia seed pudding, number 4.

Ingredients:

Include a quarter cup of chia seeds; a cup of unsweetened almond milk; and a pinch of salt.One tablespoon of honey or maple syrup; Half a teaspoon of vanilla extract; Chopped nuts or seeds (such as almonds, walnuts, or flaxseeds); Fresh fruit for topping (such as berries, sliced banana, or kiwi);

Instructions:

1. Combine the chia seeds, almond milk, honey/maple syrup, and vanilla essence in a bowl and whisk to combine. Second, put the bowl in the fridge for at least three hours, preferably overnight, so the chia seeds can soak up the liquid and thicken. Give the pudding a thorough stir before serving to make sure it's an

even consistency. Add some crunch and flavor with some chopped nuts or seeds and a serving of fresh fruit 5. Dig into your luscious chia seed pudding, loaded with healthy ingredients.

Parfait with Greek Yogurt, No. 5

Ingredients:

Greek yogurt (or a dairy-free substitute):

 1 cup• Half a cup of granola (low-sugar variety recommended)

• One-half cup of assorted berries (strawberries, blueberries, and raspberries, for example).Honey or maple syrup, 1 tbsp

• A little bit of cinnamon

Instructions:

Layer half of the Greek yogurt in a glass or bowl

2. Sprinkle a quarter of the granola over the yogurt.

Third, scatter half of the berries over the granola. Add some honey, maple syrup, and cinnamon for step 4.5 Add the remaining ingredients and repeat the layering process. Parfaits made with Greek yogurt are tasty and filling; have one right now.

These breakfast dishes will not only get your day off to a good start, but they will also help you combat melanoma. These breakfast choices are made with your healing in mind, from the antioxidant-rich berries in the smoothie to the anti-inflammatory quinoa and immune-boosting eggs in the avocado toast. Feel free to modify the recipes to suit your tastes and nutritional needs, and always check in with your doctor or a trained dietitian if you have any questions about your diet while undergoing treatment for melanoma. Throughout your path to health, you'll need to fuel your body with delicious and nourishing foods, which we'll continue to discuss in the next chapters.

Chapter 5

Delicious Noontime Treats

Lunch is a great time to refuel and reenergize for the rest of the day, and it's also a great time to eat foods that have been shown to reduce the risk of developing melanoma. These meals for lunch are not only healthy, but also delicious and filling. It doesn't matter if you're packing a lunch for the office or having a leisurely lunch at home, these meals will keep you fueled and ready to go.

Recipe: Melanoma-Fighting Salad

Ingredients:

2 cups of greens (spinach, arugula, or kale work well), 1/2 cup halved cherry tomatoes, 1/4 cup sliced cucumber thinly sliced red onion, bell peppers (red, yellow, or green), and 4 ounces of grilled chicken breast or tofu provide protein.Pumpkin seeds or nuts (such as almonds or walnuts) for crunch; 1 tablespoon of extra virgin olive oil; 1 tablespoon of balsamic vinegar; salt and pepper to taste;

Instructions:

First, assemble the salad ingredients in a large bowl: mixed greens, cherry tomatoes, cucumber, red onion, and bell peppers. Add some protein to the salad by grilling a chicken breast or some tofu. Third, make the dressing by combining the extra virgin olive oil and balsamic vinegar in a small bowl and whisking them together. Put in as much salt and pepper as you like. Toss the salad with the dressing and serve.5 For a crunchy finish and melanoma-fighting nutrients, sprinkle with pumpkin seeds or nuts. Six, eat your colorful and nutritious salad.

Stir-fried quinoa with Veggies

Ingredients: Veggies (broccoli, bell peppers, carrots, and snap peas) and quinoa (one cup cooked)• 4 ounces of protein-rich cooked shrimp, tofu, or tempeh• 2 garlic cloves, minced• 1 tablespoon gluten-free tamari or low-sodium soy sauce ingredients: 1 tbsp. sesame oil, 1/2 tsp. grated ginger, and 1 tsp. red pepper flakes (for optional extra spice).• Green onions, chopped, for garnish

Instructions:

1. In a large skillet, warm the sesame oil over medium heat. Second, stir in some garlic powder and ginger grating, and cook for 30 seconds, or until the mixture is fragrant. Third, stir-fry the medley of vegetables for about four minutes, or until they show signs of tenderness. Fourth, mix in the protein-rich cooked shrimp, tofu, or tempeh.5 Stir-fry for an extra 2 to 3 minutes, making sure everything is well-mixed, after which you may add the cooked quinoa. Scatter

the stir-fry with the scallions and toss with the low-sodium soy sauce or tamari.7 Season with red pepper flakes to taste if you like things spicy. Chopped green onions add a burst of freshness; use them as a garnish in step 8.9 Enjoy the delicious and filling tastes of your quinoa and veggie stir-fry while it's still hot.

Salad with lentils and sweet potatoes

Ingredients:

In addition to 2 medium sweet potatoes, 1 cup of cooked green or brown lentils, and 1/4 cup of crumbled feta cheese (optional), you'll need the following ingredients.Ingredients: 1/4 cup chopped fresh parsley 2 tbsp extra virgin olive oil 1 tbsp balsamic vinegar salt and pepper to taste optional smoked paprika

Instructions:

1. Set oven temperature to 400 degrees Fahrenheit (200 degrees Celsius). Dice the sweet potatoes and place them on a baking sheet; then, if using, sprinkle them with salt, pepper, and smoky paprika. Coat toss. Until soft and slightly caramelized, roast the sweet potatoes for 20-25 minutes. Mix the cooked lentils and roasted

sweet potatoes in a large salad dish. Fifth, dress the salad with the remaining olive oil and balsamic vinegar

6. If using, sprinkle in some crumbled feta cheese and fresh chopped parsley.

7. Toss everything together so that the dressing covers all the ingredients.

8. If necessary, add salt and pepper to taste.

9. During lunch, offer your guests your sweet potato and lentil salad.

Wrapped in the Mediterranean

Ingredients:

Include: • 1 whole-grain wrap or tortilla (gluten-free version available if necessary);• 3 ounces of grilled chicken breast, falafel, or roasted chickpeas (for protein) • 2 tablespoons of hummus (store-bought or homemade)Include: 1/2 cup of greens (arugula or spinach work well), 1/4 cup of cucumber slices, 1/4 cup of cherry tomatoes, 1/4 cup of Kalamata olive slices, and 2 tablespoons of crumbled feta cheese (if desired).• Tzatziki sauce or Greek yogurt for drizzling (optional)

Instructions:

First, on a plate or other clean surface, spread out the whole-grain wrap or tortilla.

Second, smear the wrap with a lot of hummus. Then, pile on some protein in the form of grilled chicken, falafel, or roasted chickpeas.

 Third, top with a variety of greens, cucumber slices, cherry tomatoes, and Kalamata olives

 5. If preferred, top the vegetables with crumbled feta cheese. To enhance the flavor and smoothness, step six is to drizzle tzatziki sauce or Greek yogurt over the ingredients. Seven, roll the wrap up tightly, tucking the sides in as you go. Cut on the diagonal for a speedy meal.9 Have a delicious and filling lunch with your wrap, which was inspired by the cuisine of the Mediterranean.

Warming Lentil Soup

Ingredients:

1 cup of rinsed and drained dried green or brown lentils; 6 cups of low-sodium vegetable or chicken broth; 1 chopped onion; 2 carrots; 2 celery stalks; 2 minced garlic cloves; 1 teaspoon of olive oil; 1 teaspoon of ground cumin; 1/2 teaspoon of ground turmeric; 1/2 teaspoon of smoked paprika; salt and pepper to taste; fresh lemon juice for garnish (optional); chopped fresh parsley (optional).

Instructions:

To begin, heat the olive oil in a large soup pot over medium heat. Then, after about 5 minutes of sautéing, add the chopped onion, carrots, and celery and stir. Finally, after 2 minutes of sautéing, add the minced garlic, ground cumin, ground turmeric, and smoked paprika and stir until aromatic. Fourth, after washing the lentils, put them in a pot with some low-sodium chicken or veggie broth.

To taste, add salt and pepper and then step 5.

To cook the lentils, you should bring the mixture to a boil, then reduce the heat and let it simmer for 25-30 minutes.

6. Check the seasoning and make any necessary changes.

7. If wanted, serve the hearty lentil soup hot, topped with a squeeze of fresh lemon juice and some chopped fresh parsley.

These tasty lunch ideas are also loaded with elements known to inhibit the growth of melanoma. Each dish, from the cheery Melanoma-Busting Salad to the soothing Hearty Lentil Soup, is formulated to supply vital nutrients to help you feel your best as you fight melanoma. Feel free to modify the recipes to suit your tastes and nutritional needs, and always check in with your doctor or a qualified dietitian if you have any questions about your diet. Throughout your path to health, you'll need to fuel your body with delicious and nourishing foods, which we'll continue to discuss in the next chapters.

Chapter 6

Dinner for Health

As the day comes to a close, dinner is a great time to relax, fuel your body, and check that you're getting everything you need to thrive as you fight melanoma. The components in these meal recipes were chosen specifically for their ability to combat melanoma. We've got you covered for dinner with everything from hearty stews to delectable grilled foods.

Citrus-Glazed Grilled Salmon

Ingredients:• 2 salmon fillets (about 6-8 ounces each)2 tablespoons honey or maple syrup 1 tablespoon olive oil 2 minced garlic cloves Zest and juice of 1 lemon Zest and juice of 1 orange garnish with fresh herbs (such chopped parsley or dill) and season with salt and pepper to suit.

Instructions:

First, make the citrus glaze by combining the following ingredients in a bowl: lemon zest, lemon juice, orange zest, orange juice, honey/maple syrup, olive oil, chopped garlic, salt, and pepper. Second, on a wide, shallow dish, cover the salmon fillets with half of the citrus glaze. They need at least 15 minutes of marinating time. Third, have a medium-high flame going in your grill. Cook the salmon fillets on a hot grill for 3 to 4 minutes per side, or until they are opaque throughout and flake readily when tested with a fork. Fifth, use the remaining citrus glaze to coat the salmon and grill it for the last minute. Take the salmon from the grill and sprinkle some herbs on top. Seven, accompany your citrus-glazed grilled salmon with a side salad or your preferred vegetables.

Second, a Chickpea and Quinoa Stew

Ingredients:

4 cups of low-sodium vegetable broth; 1 teaspoon of olive oil; 1 teaspoon of ground cumin; 1/2 teaspoon of ground paprika; salt and pepper to taste; chopped fresh cilantro for garnish (optional); 1 cup of cooked quinoa; 1 can (15 oz) of chickpeas; 1 can (15 oz) of diced tomatoes; 1 chopped onion; 2 minced garlic cloves; 2 carrots; 2 celery stalks; 1 diced bell pepper (red

Instructions:

To begin, heat the olive oil in a large soup pot over medium heat. Next, throw in some chopped veggies like onions, garlic, carrots, celery, and peppers. To soften the vegetables, sauté them for around 5 minutes. After 2 minutes of sautéing, add the ground cumin and paprika and stir until fragrant.4 Put in the canned tomatoes, canned chickpeas, and quinoa. Fifth, add the sodium-reduced vegetable broth. Add salt and pepper to taste, then number 6. Until the veggies are soft and the flavors have blended, simmer the mixture for 20-25 minutes after bringing it to a boil.8. Give it a try and season it to your liking.9 - If you like, sprinkle some chopped fresh cilantro on top of your hot quinoa and chickpea stew.

Salad with Grilled Veggies and Lentils

Ingredients:

1 cup of rinsed and drained green or brown lentils 2 cups of grilled vegetables (such as zucchini, eggplant, bell peppers, and asparagus) 1/4 cup of crumbled feta cheese (optional) 2 tablespoons of extra virgin olive oil 1 tablespoon of balsamic vinegar 1 minced clove of garlic Salt and pepper to taste Garnish with fresh basil leaves

Instructions:

First, put the lentils in a pot and add enough water to cover them by an inch. Simmer for 15-

20 minutes until the lentils are soft but not mushy, after which they should be brought to a boil again. Rinse them under cold water and set them aside to cool. Second, have a medium-high flame going in your grill. Third, cook the veggies until soft and marked with grill marks, about 5 to 7 minutes per side. Fourth, toss the grilled veggies and cooked lentils in a big salad dish.5 Make the dressing by combining the extra virgin olive oil, balsamic vinegar, minced garlic, salt, and pepper in a small bowl and whisking until smooth. Toss the salad with the dressing and step #6.7 For extra richness, you can top it with crumbled feta cheese. Put a few fresh basil leaves over top for extra flavor. Nine, for a healthy and filling dinner, serve your grilled veggie and lentil salad.

Quinoa with Lemon Herb Chicken

Ingredients:

One cup of cooked quinoa One lemon's worth of zested and juice Two boneless, skinless chicken breasts, each weighing in at 6-8 ounces• 2 garlic cloves, mincedUse 1 tablespoon of olive oil, 2 tablespoons of fresh herbs (such as chopped parsley, thyme, or rosemary), salt, pepper, and lemon wedges to season to taste.

Instructions:

To make the marinade, combine the lemon zest, lemon juice, garlic, herbs, olive oil, salt, and pepper in a bowl and stir together. In a shallow dish, lay the chicken breasts and cover them with the marinade. They need at least 15 minutes of marinating time. Third, get a grill or grill pan nice and hot on medium heat. For 6-7 minutes per side, or until the chicken is fully cooked and grill marks appear, place the chicken breasts on a preheated grill. Reheat the quinoa while you grill the chicken. Place the grilled chicken with lemon herb sauce on a bed of quinoa and serve. Seven, for a zesty citrus kick, top with lemon wedges. Eight, savor the delectable meal that is also high in protein.

Five. Spaghetti Squash Loaded with Vegetables

Ingredients:

2 cups of halved cherry tomatoes 1 diced bell pepper (red, yellow, or green) 1 diced zucchini 1 diced onion 2 minced cloves of garlic 2

tablespoons of olive oil 1 teaspoon of Italian seasoning salt and pepper to taste and some fresh basil leaves for garnish

Instructions:

First, have a 375°F (190°C) oven ready. Second, remove the spaghetti squash's seeds by slicing it in half lengthwise.3 Arrange the squash halves on a baking sheet, cut side up. Season with salt and pepper and drizzle with olive oil. When the squash is delicate enough to be scraped into spaghetti-like strands with a fork, it has roasted long enough in the preheated oven (approximately 45 minutes).5. Preheat a big skillet with the olive oil over medium heat while you roast the squash.

6. Put in some onion and garlic and cook for a couple of minutes until they start to release their aroma.

Dice up some bell pepper and zucchini and add them to the skillet. Saute for another 5 to 7 minutes, or until the vegetables begin to soften.

7. Add the cherry tomatoes, cut in half, and Italian seasoning and stir. To heat the tomatoes, continue to sauté for another 2–3 minutes.

To taste, add salt and pepper to the ingredients in step 8.

9.Roast the spaghetti squash until tender, and then use a fork to scrape the meat into strands.

Add the sautéed vegetable combination to the vegetable-packed spaghetti squash and serve.

Twelve, for an extra kick of flavor, top with a few basil leaves.

Thirteen, have a healthy and colorful meal.

These scrumptious main dish recipes also happen to be melanoma-prevention powerhouses. Each recipe, from the grilled salmon with citrus glaze to the substantial quinoa and chickpea stew, has been created to give you the nutrition you need to fight melanoma. Feel free to modify the recipes to suit your tastes and nutritional needs, and always check in with your doctor or a qualified dietitian if you have any questions about your diet. Throughout your path to health, you'll need to fuel your body with delicious and nourishing foods, which we'll continue to discuss in the next chapters.

Certainly! In a cookbook dedicated to the treatment of melanoma, the next 800 words cover the topic of "Snacks and Sides"

Chapter7

Additional Dishes

Enjoyable and nourishing snacks can be incorporated into a melanoma-fighting diet. It's a chance to get in some extra nutrients between meals, curb hunger pangs, and maintain your energy levels. In this chapter, we'll investigate many nutritious snack options and accompaniments that not only taste good but also contain melanoma-preventive substances.

1. Guacamole that Fights Skin Cancer

Ingredients: Two ripe avocados, peeled and pitted; one small red onion, finely chopped; one to two cloves of garlic, minced; two small tomatoes, diced; the juice of one lime; one-fourth cup of fresh cilantro, chopped; salt and pepper to taste; red pepper flakes (optional, for added heat); a variety of raw vegetables for dipping (carrots, cucumbers, bell peppers, etc.); and whole-grain tortilla chips for scooping.

Instructions:1. Put the ripe avocados in a basin and mash them with a fork. Then, throw in some fresh cilantro, tomato cubes, minced garlic, and finely sliced red onion. Add the juice of one lime and stir everything together. To taste, add salt and pepper.5 Red pepper flakes can be used for spiciness if desired. Blend the guacamole until the ingredients are evenly distributed and the consistency is creamy (step 6).To make a healthy and filling snack, combine your Melanoma-Busting Guacamole with fresh veggie sticks or whole-grain tortilla chips.

Chickpeas, roasted

Ingredients:

1 can of chickpeas (15 ounces), drained and rinsed; 1 tablespoon of olive oil; 1 teaspoon of smoked paprika; 1/2 teaspoon of crushed cumin; 1/2 teaspoon of garlic powder pepper and salt to taste

Instructions:

1. Set oven temperature to 400 degrees Fahrenheit (200 degrees Celsius). The chickpeas should be washed, drained, and dried with a clean dish towel before proceeding. Mix the chickpeas, olive oil, smoked paprika, ground cumin, garlic powder, salt, and pepper in a bowl. Fourth, spread down a single layer of chickpeas on a baking sheet 5. Roast in the preheated oven

until the chickpeas are crispy and golden brown, about 25-30 minutes, stirring the pan regularly to ensure equal cooking. Take them out of the oven, and set them to cool for a few minutes.7 Put those protein-packed roasted chickpeas to good use as a crispy snack.

3 Dip with Cucumbers and Greek Yogurt

Ingredients:

In a bowl, combine 1 cup Greek yogurt (or a dairy-free substitute), 1 minced garlic clove, and 1 cup of grated and squeezed cucumber.Ingredients: • 1 tablespoon of minced fresh dill • 1 tablespoon of lemon juice include: • Fresh vegetable sticks (such as carrots, celery, and cucumber) for dipping; • Salt and pepper to taste

Instructions:

Step 1: After grating the cucumber, squeeze out as much liquid as possible using a clean dish towel. Grate the cucumber and place it in a bowl with the Greek yogurt, garlic, dill, lemon juice, and minced garlic. To taste, add salt and pepper. 4. Mix vigorously until all ingredients are incorporated 5. Chill the dip in the fridge for at least 30 minutes before serving so that the flavors can combine. For a healthy and protein-packed snack, try serving Cucumber and Greek Yogurt Dip with raw veggie sticks.

4. Hummus and a Rainbow Platter of Veggies

Ingredients:

Bell peppers, cherry tomatoes, carrots, cucumber, and sugar snap peas are just a few examples of the brightly colored fresh vegetables that are available.• Hummus, either premade or from scratch• Garnishing herbs (such as parsley or chives)

Instructions:

First, clean the raw vegetables and cut them into sticks or small chunks. Make a rainbow with the multicolored vegetables on a serving dish.3. Center the dish with a bowl of hummus. To improve the taste and appearance, garnish with fresh herbs. Five, for a healthy and colorful snack or side dish, serve a rainbow vegetable platter with hummus.

6. Pomegranate and quinoa salad

Ingredients:

Two cups of cooked quinoa, cooled; one cup of pomegranate seeds; half a cup of chopped cucumber; half a cup of chopped red bell pepper; a quarter cup of chopped fresh mint leaves; the juice of one lemon; two teaspoons of extra virgin olive oil; salt and pepper to taste; crumbled feta cheese (optional).

Instructions:

Then, mix the quinoa, pomegranate seeds, cucumber, red bell pepper, and fresh mint leaves in a big bowl after they have cooled.2. Make the dressing by combining the lemon juice, extra virgin olive oil, salt, and pepper in a small bowl and whisking until smooth. Toss the quinoa salad with the dressing to coat. You can make it more creamier by topping it with crumbled feta cheese.5 As a refreshing and antioxidant-rich side dish or snack, serve your quinoa salad with pomegranate seeds.

Sixth, Sweet Potato Fries, Baked

Ingredients:

Fries made with 2 medium sweet potatoes, peeled and sliced into fries shapes, seasoned with smoky paprika, garlic powder, and olive oil.Ingredients: Onion powder, 1/2 teaspoon pepper and salt to taste

Instructions:

To begin, prepare a baking dish by preheating the oven to 425 degrees Fahrenheit (220 degrees Celsius). Place the sweet potato fries in a bowl and add the olive oil, smoked paprika, garlic powder, onion powder, salt, and pepper. Place the fries in a single layer on a baking sheet and bake for 30 minutes. To make the fries crispy and gently browned, put them in an oven at 400 degrees for 25-30 minutes and flip them halfway through baking.5 Get them out of the oven and let them cool down a little. Baked sweet potato fries are a delicious and healthy addition to any meal or snack.

7. Berry Yogurt Parfait with Almonds

Ingredients:

Greek yogurt (or a dairy-free substitute): 1 cup includes: 1/2 cup of mixed berries (blueberries, strawberries, raspberries), 2 tablespoons of sliced almonds, and 1/2 cup of Greek yogurt. Honey or maple syrup, 1 tablespoon; cinnamon, to taste

Instructions:

Layer half of the Greek yogurt in a glass or bowl. Then, place half of the berry mixture on top of the yogurt. Three, top the berries with chopped almonds. Sweeten with honey or maple syrup and cinnamon, then serve.5 Add the remaining ingredients and repeat the layering process. 6 Eat your antioxidant-rich Berry and Almond Yogurt Parfait as a pleasant snack or side dish. These dishes for snacks and sides not only taste great, but also use elements known to inhibit the growth of melanoma. Each recipe, from the zesty Melanoma-Busting Guacamole to the crisp Roasted Chickpeas, is a delicious way to boost your health and wellness on your melanoma journey. Feel free to modify the recipes to suit your tastes and nutritional needs, and always check in with your doctor or a qualified dietitian if you have any questions about your diet. Throughout your path to health, you'll need to fuel your body with delicious and nourishing foods, which we'll continue to discuss in the next chapters.

<h1 style="text-align:center">Chapter 8</h1>

<h2 style="text-align:center">Benefiting from Dessert</h2>

Who says you can't eat something sweet on a diet that helps prevent melanoma? In this section, we'll talk about sweets that can both satisfy your sweet taste and improve your health. These sweet treats are healthy for you because they are made with antioxidant- and vitamin- and mineral-rich components.

1. Fruit and dark chocolate parfait

Ingredients:

• One-half cup of Greek yogurt (or dairy-free equivalent)

Crumbled dark chocolate (2 squares, 70% cocoa or higher)

• One-half cup of assorted berries (strawberries, blueberries, etc.)

• Sweeten to taste with honey or maple syrup, if desired (one tablespoon).

• Mint leaves, fresh for garnishing (but not required)

Instructions:

Half of the Greek yogurt should be layered in a glass or bowl.

Sprinkle the yogurt with half of the chopped dark chocolate.

Sprinkle a quarter of the berry mixture over the chocolate.

Honey or maple syrup can be used to provide sweetness.

Add the remaining ingredients in a second layer.

To add a blast of fresh taste, garnish with mint leaves.

The Dark Chocolate Berry Parfait is a healthy and satisfying dessert option.

2. Banana and almond butter bites

Ingredients:

• One banana, peeled and sliced thinly

Two tablespoons of almond butter (or your preferred nut or seed butter)

• 2 tbsp of shredded coconut, preferably sweetened

Chia seeds, 1 tbsp

Add 1/2 tsp. of cinnamon powder

• Raw honey (or maple syrup) to drizzle (optional)

Instructions:

Cover each banana slice with almond butter.

Combine shredded coconut, chia seeds, and cinnamon in a wide, shallow bowl.

Coat each banana round with almond butter, then dip it into the coconut-chia mixture and gently push it to adhere.

Arrange the banana rounds in a single layer on a dish or tray.

Raw honey or maple syrup can be used as a sweetener if desired.

Put in the fridge for at least 15 minutes to chill before serving.

These bites of banana and almond butter are a healthy and delicious dessert option.

3. Fruit with Chia Pudding

Ingredients:

Chia seeds, about a quarter cup

• 1 cup of almond milk (or your preferred milk, if sweetened)

• One-half cup of assorted berries (strawberries, blueberries, etc.)

• Sweeten to taste with honey or maple syrup, if desired (one tablespoon).

• Mint leaves, fresh for garnishing (but not required)

Instructions:

Combine chia seeds and almond milk in a bowl and mix well.

Allow the chia seeds to absorb the liquid and thicken in the fridge for at least 3 hours or overnight before serving.

Give the chia pudding a quick swirl before serving to make sure the consistency is uniform.

Lightly mash the mixed berries with a fork to release some juices in a separate bowl.

Put the chia pudding in the bottom of a bowl or glass and top it with the mashed berries.

You can sweeten it up with honey or maple syrup if you like.

Use mint leaves as a garnish for a burst of brightness.

Chia seed and berry pudding is a delicious dish that is high in antioxidants and creamy to boot.

4. Yogurt with fruity bark, frozen.

Ingredients:

Greek yogurt (or a dairy-free substitute): 1 cup

• One cup of assorted berries (strawberries, blueberries, and raspberries, for example).

Honey or maple syrup, 1 tbsp

Chopped nuts (such as almonds, walnuts, or pistachios)—2 tablespoons

• A little bit of cinnamon

Instructions:

Greek yogurt and honey or maple syrup should be mixed together thoroughly in a bowl.

Prepare parchment paper on a baking pan.

Evenly coat the parchment paper with the sweetened yogurt.

1. Sprinkle the yogurt with the chopped nuts, mixed berries, and cinnamon.

2. Yogurt bark needs to be frozen for at least two hours.

3. Take it out of the freezer and smash it into bits.

4. Make a healthy and delicious dessert with your Frozen Yogurt and Berry Bark.

5. Apples in cinnamon and walnuts, baked in the oven.

Ingredients:

• Two peeled and halved apples

1) One-fourth cup of chopped walnuts

• Cinnamon, ground, one teaspoon

Honey or maple syrup, 1 tbsp

• Vanilla or Greek yogurt, to serve (optional).

Instructions:

1. Start by preheating the oven to 375 degrees Fahrenheit (190 degrees Celsius).

2. Combine walnut pieces, cinnamon, and sweetener (honey or maple syrup) in a small bowl.

3. Arrange the apple halves on a baking sheet, and cut side up.

5. For 20-25 minutes in a warm oven, or until apples are soft and beginning to caramelize.

6. Take them out of the oven and reduce the heat by a few degrees.

7. Warm and cozy, your Baked Apples with Cinnamon and Walnuts will be the perfect end to a meal.

8. Greek yogurt or vanilla yogurt, if preferred, can be used as a topping.

6. Chocolate-Avocado Mousse

Ingredients:

• 2 ripe avocados, peeled and seeded

Ingredients: •

 1/4 cup cocoa powder (unsweetened)

• One-fourth cup of maple syrup or honey

• Vanilla extract, 1 teaspoon

• A dash of pepper

• Garnish with fresh berries (strawberries, raspberries, etc.)

Instructions:

1. Blend or process the ripe avocados with the unsweetened cocoa powder, honey/maple syrup,

vanilla essence, and a sprinkling of salt until smooth.

2. Scrape down the sides of the blender as needed and blend until the mixture is smooth and creamy.

3. If extra sweetness is wanted, add some honey or maple syrup and taste again.

The avocado chocolate mousse should be divided amongst serving dishes or glasses.

5. Serve after chilling in the fridge for at least half an hour.

6. Use fresh berries as a garnish to add a blast of flavor and healthy antioxidants.

7. This Avocado Chocolate Mousse is a decadent treat that won't leave you feeling guilty.

7. Oatmeal Cookies with Dried Berries

Ingredients:

1.25 ounces of chia seeds

The equivalent of half a cup of whole wheat flour (or gluten-free flour mix)

• A quarter cup of nut or seed butter (we used almond)

• One-fourth cup of maple syrup or honey

• Mixed berries (blueberries, raspberries, strawberries), about a quarter cup, cut if very large

• One-fourth cup of natural apple sauce

• Vanilla extract, 1 teaspoon

Add 1/2 tsp. of cinnamon powder

In a small bowl, whisk together:

• A dash of pepper

Instructions:

1. Get the oven up to temperature, preferably 350 degrees Fahrenheit (175 degrees Celsius).

2. Mix together the oats, flour, honey or maple syrup, berries, applesauce (without added sugar), vanilla extract, cinnamon, baking powder, and

salt in a large basin. The ingredients should be mixed until they stick together.

3. Use a spoon to place cookie dough onto a baking sheet covered in parchment paper.

4. Put the cookie dough into an oven that has been prepared to 350 degrees and bake for 12 to 15 minutes.

5. Take them out of the oven and cool them on a rack.

6. Your chewy and fiber-rich Berry and Oatmeal Cookies are ready to be devoured.

8. Chia Popsicles with Mango Puree and Coconut Milk

Ingredients:

• Two cups of diced, peeled, ripe mango

Coconut Milk, One Cup

Chia seeds, enough for 2 tablespoons

• Sweeten to taste with honey or maple syrup, if desired (one tablespoon).

Instructions:

1. Blend or process the mango cubes with the coconut milk. Throw everything in the blender and puree until silky.

2. If more or less sweetness is wanted, try adding honey or maple syrup and tasting again.

3. Add chia seeds and combine thoroughly.

4. Fill popsicle molds with the mango and coconut mixture.

5.Put the popsicles in the freezer for at least four hours, preferably longer.

6.Take them out of the freezer and you'll have a tropical and delicious dessert.

These dessert recipes will not only satisfy your sweet tooth, but will also help you maintain your health as you fight melanoma. Each dessert is a delicious way to reward yourself while sticking to a melanoma-prevention diet, from the Dark Chocolate and Berry Parfait to the Berry and Oatmeal Cookies. Feel free to modify the recipes to suit your tastes and nutritional needs, and always check in with your doctor or a qualified dietitian if you have any questions about your diet. Throughout your path to health, you'll need to fuel your body with delicious and nourishing foods, which we'll continue to discuss in the next chapters.

Chapter 9

Drinks that Heal

The drinks you select can play a significant part in your quest for general health as you battle melanoma. Beverages not only help you stay hydrated, but they can also provide you with melanoma-fighting chemicals. In this section, we'll take a look at some drinks that can help you stay hydrated while also providing beneficial nutrients and antioxidants for your body.

1. Elixir de Thé Vert

The high levels of catechin antioxidants found in green tea have earned it much praise for improving health. Green tea's antioxidants are worth considering if you spend time outdoors in the sun, as they may help prevent skin damage and cancer.

Ingredients:

• 1 sachet of green tea

• 1 mug of simmering water

• Sweeten to taste with honey, if desired (one teaspoon).

• Optional (but highly recommended) fresh lemon juice squeezed

• Mint leaves (optional, but much recommended)

Instructions:

1. Get a cup and drop it in the green tea bag.

2. Use a hot water kettle to brew your tea.

3. Allow it to steep for three to five minutes.

4. Take out the tea bag and flavor it with honey, lemon juice, or mint if you like.

5. Green tea elixir is an anti-inflammatory and antioxidant-rich drink.

2. Water with Refreshing Cucumbers and Lemon

Cucumber and lemon water are a delicious way to stay hydrated while also adding a blast of flavor and some important vitamins to your day.

Ingredients:

• Half of a cucumber, sliced very thinly

• One lemon, sliced very thinly

• 8 cups (or a pitcher) of water

• Mint leaves (for flavor and optional freshness)

Instructions:

1. In a pitcher of water, float the cucumber and lemon slices.

2.Allow flavors to blend by chilling for at least an hour before serving.

3. Your pleasant and hydrating Cucumber and Lemon Water is ready to be served.

4. Fresh mint leaves make a great garnish.

3. Lattes with Golden Milk

The anti-inflammatory and possible immune-enhancing qualities of turmeric (the "golden spice"). This delicious golden milk latte is a soothing way to include turmeric in your diet.

Ingredients:

One cup of milk (regular or almond)

• One-half teaspoon of turmeric powder

• One-fourth of a teaspoon of cinnamon powder

• A dash of black pepper (which aids in the absorption of turmeric)

• Sweeten to taste with honey or maple syrup, if desired (one teaspoon).

Instructions:

1. Milk should be heated over low heat in a small saucepan.

2. Add a dash of black pepper and stir in ground turmeric, cinnamon, ginger, and other spices.

3. Stirring occasionally, heat the mixture until it is hot but not boiling.

4. Add honey or maple syrup for sweetness if you like.

5. Warm up with a mug of Golden Milk Latte, a drink touted for its anti-inflammatory and soothing properties.

4. Smoothie Made with Antioxidant-Rich Berries

Antioxidants found in abundance in berries have been shown to aid in skin protection and general health. Smoothies like this one made with fresh berries are a tasty and healthy way to add more berries to your diet.

Ingredients:

• One-half cup of a variety of berries (strawberries, blueberries, etc.)

Banana, Half a

• One-half cup of Greek yogurt (or dairy-free equivalent)

• Half a cup of milk (regular or soy-based).

• Sweeten to taste with honey or maple syrup, if desired (one tablespoon).

Ingredients: 12 tsp. vanilla extract

Instructions:

1. Blend together some mixed berries, a banana, Greek yogurt, milk, some honey or maple syrup, and some vanilla extract.

2. Mix until the mixture is silky.

3. Fill a glass with your Antioxidant-Rich Berry Smoothie and sip on something delicious while getting a healthy dose of antioxidants.

5. Infusion of Watermelon and Mint

As a bonus, watermelon contains the antioxidant lycopene, which may help prevent sun damage to the skin. Stay cool and hydrated with this infusion of watermelon and mint.

Ingredients:

• Two cups of diced fresh watermelon

Leaves of fresh mint

• 8 cups (or a pitcher) of water

Instructions:

1. Watermelon cubes and mint leaves can be added to a pitcher of water for a refreshing drink.

2. Let the flavors meld in the fridge for at least an hour before serving.

3. Make a refreshing and hydrating drink using watermelon and mint and serve it to your guests.

4. Freshen it up with some additional mint leaves and serve.

6. Carrot and Beet Juice

Nitrates, which are abundant in beets, have been shown to benefit blood flow and heart function. Incorporating these colorful root veggies into your diet need not be a chore with this delicious beet and carrot juice.

Ingredients:

• Two beets, roughly sliced and peeled

• 2 peeled and sliced carrots

• One apple, peeled, cored, and cut

• Fresh ginger, cut into 1-inch pieces

• Peeled lemon half (12)

• An optional dash of salt

Instructions:

1. Use a juicer to process the diced beets, carrots, apple, ginger, and lemon.

2. Season with salt, to taste, if you want.

3. Be proud to offer your guests a drink that is both delicious and healthy.

7. Pineapple and coconut water slushie

Coconut water is an electrolyte-rich natural beverage that can aid with hydration, and pineapple adds a tropical flavor and critical nutrients.

Ingredients:

Coconut water, one cup's worth

Fresh or frozen pineapple pieces, 1/2 cup

One lime's juice

• Sweeten to taste with honey or maple syrup, if desired (one tablespoon).

Cubed ice

Instructions:

1. Blend together ice cubes, coconut water, frozen pineapple chunks, lime juice, and honey or maple syrup (to taste).

2. Get it nice and icy by blending it.

3. Give your guests a taste of the tropics with your Coconut Water and Pineapple Cooler.

8. Hibiscus Herbal Tea

The antioxidant and heart-health advantages of hibiscus tea are well-documented, and the tea's bright hue is a bonus. Caffeine-free and delicious, this herbal hibiscus tea can be enjoyed at any time of the day.

Ingredients:

• 1 tbsp of dried hibiscus petals or 1 hibiscus tea bag

• 1 mug of simmering water

• Sweeten to taste with honey or maple syrup, if desired (one teaspoon).

• Optional (but highly recommended) fresh lemon juice squeezed

Instructions:

1. You can use a tea bag or some dried hibiscus blossoms to make a hibiscus drink.

2. Douse the tea with steaming water.

3. Brew for 5 minutes.

4. To get rid of the petals, either take out the tea bag or drain the tea.

5. You may sweeten it up with some honey, maple syrup, and fresh lemon juice.

6. Herbal Hibiscus Tea is a delicious way to get your daily dose of antioxidants.

In addition to helping you stay hydrated, the components in these drinks have been shown to inhibit the growth of melanoma cells. Each drink offers a delightful and nourishing alternative to boost your well-being during your melanoma journey, from the antioxidant-rich Green Tea Elixir to the moisturizing Cucumber and Lemon Water. Feel free to modify the recipes to suit your tastes and nutritional needs, and always check in with your doctor or a qualified dietitian if you have any questions about your diet. Throughout your path to health, you'll need to fuel your body with delicious and nourishing foods, which we'll continue to discuss in the next chapters.

Conclusion

When you're done with this Melanoma Cancer Diet Cookbook, we hope you'll have found more than simply a tasty assortment of dishes; you'll have uncovered a potent resource for nourishing your body, bolstering your health, and maximizing your well-being as you fight this disease. In this book, we've covered a wide variety of meals, snacks, sides, desserts, and drinks, all of which are designed to give you the nutrients and antioxidants you need to combat melanoma.

Diet plays an important role in your overall health, but your path to well-being is complex and very personal. We've done our best to give you recipes that are not only healthy and tasty but also adaptable to your specific dietary requirements. To make these recipes work for you, we recommend consulting with your healthcare provider or a qualified dietitian.

Keeping to a diet that helps fight melanoma is only one part of the battle. These recipes should be used in conjunction with your doctor's advice and prescribed treatment. In your fight against melanoma, your medical team is your first and most important line of defense.

While the food you eat is certainly a significant part of your journey, there are many other aspects of self-care that deserve your attention as well. Take care of your mental and emotional health by managing stress, spending time with positive people, staying physically active, and eating a healthy diet. These factors, along with careful dietary considerations, can help you recover much more quickly.

The fight against melanoma will be difficult, but you will face it with courage, strength, and optimism. Preparing and enjoying a meal from this cookbook can be a daily reminder of your commitment to a happy, healthy lifestyle. Thank God for another day, and keep in mind that you can influence your future by the decisions you make today.

We hope that you will soon be on the road to recovery. The recipes and information herein are offered to you as a source of solace, inspiration, and strength on your journey. You may count on the help of friends, family, medical professionals, and other resources while you go through this process.

Be resilient, have an optimistic outlook, and relish each step along the way to a better, healthier tomorrow.